THE TUMMY TRIMMER PRIMER

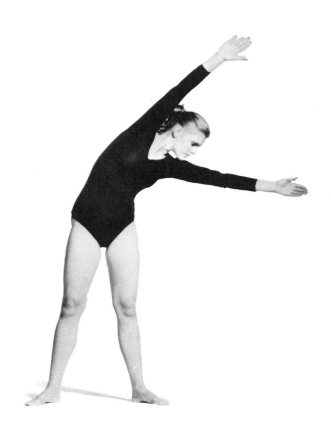

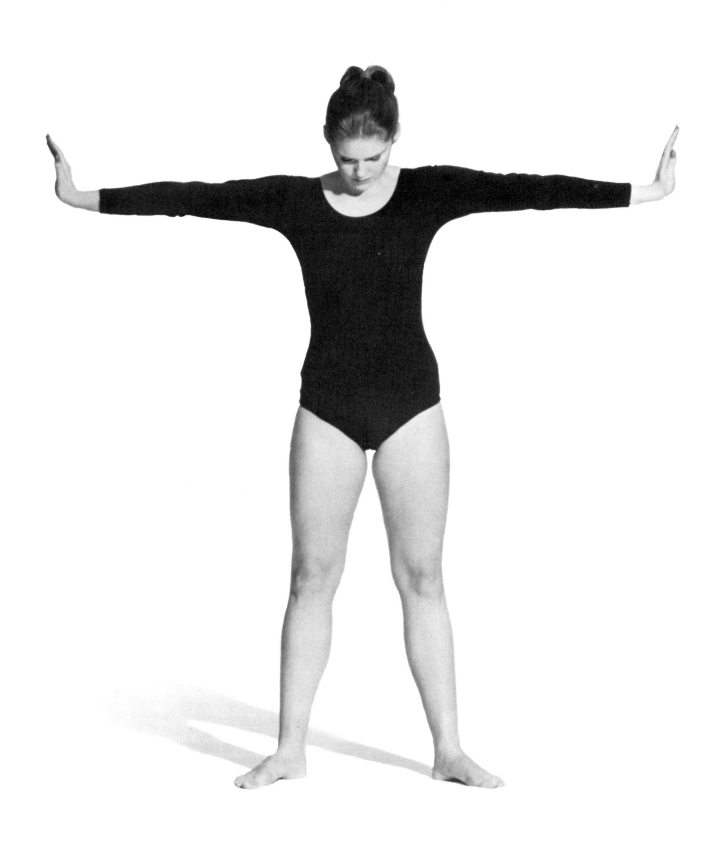

THE TUMMY TRIMMER PRIMER

by Ann Smith

GROSSET & DUNLAP
PUBLISHERS · NEW YORK
A Filmways Company

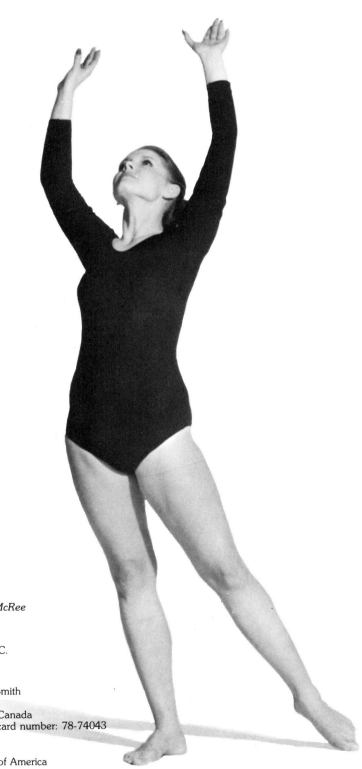

Designed by Giorgetta Bell McRee

photographs by
MORT ENGEL STUDIO, INC.
NEW YORK CITY

Published simultaneously in Canada
Library of Congress catalog card number: 78-74043
ISBN 0−448−16293−8
First printing 1979
Printed in the United States of America

Contents

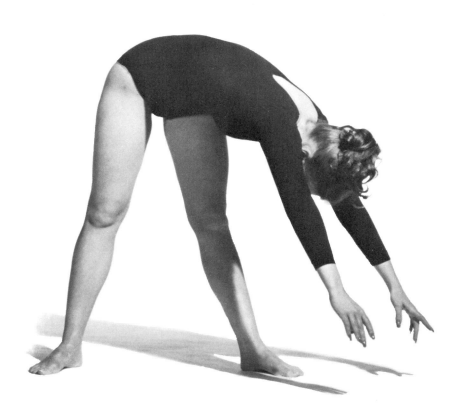

Introduction

For reasons of both health and vanity, the area of the body that causes the most anguish and discontent for both men and women is the stomach/hip section. Most people are unhappy with the size, protrusion, and excess weight they carry there, and they'd like to be rid of them.

I'm sure that many fat-tummied, huge-hipped people frequently try various ways to get rid of their stomachs, but without much success. Otherwise, there wouldn't be so many diet and exercise books on the market, each one holding out new hope and promising great things.

But even if you spent all your free time exercising and stopped eating, you still might be pathetically out of shape. There's got to be another answer.

There is. And it's so obviously based on simple logic and common sense that after reading this book you'll wonder why you didn't think of it yourself.

You probably don't need a technical explanation of the muscles involved and their relation to specific visceral activity to realize what you're doing to yourself physically by walking around with a fat tummy. You're already unhappy about your condition and aren't interested in whether the protrusion has stretched and made ineffective the *rectus abdominis*, the *transversus abdominis*, or the *internal* and *external obliques*.

You just want to make your stomach smaller. You want to be able to pull it in and make it flat. You want to have narrower hips. You want to look better and feel better.

That's not hard to do if you understand how you got out of shape, change the pattern, and then restore yourself with a simple set of exercises that will lift, realign, flatten, and maintain your body the way you want it to be—beautifully proportionate and healthy.

The Tummy Trimmer Primer was written to answer the demand for an exercise routine that will really do the job. It's designed to take you back to the beginning of the subject of exercise and build on a few basic rules of body nature so that you can expand your working knowledge of exercise and reach the ultimate goal—a flat stomach and narrow hips.

This primer has been pared down to cover only exercises that will do the most dramatic job on your stomach and hips as easily, efficiently, and quickly as possible. Of course, in the process, the rest of the body will be proportioned and restored too. The exercises can be done by both men and women. Performed slowly and properly, they are effective for people of any age.

As you read the book, learning and doing the exercises at the same time, you'll understand that the whole subject centers on one concept—an uplifted body position. Once your body senses learn that, you'll be able to walk around free of an unsightly stomach and large hips once and for all. I'm sure you'll be a lot healthier and happier.

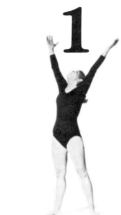

How You Get a Tummy and How to Get Rid of It

Animals at birth move in the exact structural position that they maintain through life, in movement and at rest. People must develop from a fetal position the ability to sit, crawl, and stand. When awake we are vertical; at rest we change our skeletal position to horizontal. Considering all the growth processes we go through to reach full physical development, and the daily skeletal adjustments we must make between vertical and horizontal positions, we really do quite well.

But even so, the human body is always vulnerable to a gradual downward shifting of weight—from poor posture positions, fatigue, laziness, emotional states that make us physically droop, and the general physical-emotional responsibility of holding everything up.

As we are constantly changing the vertical balance of our positions within various daily routines, these changing positions become our postures—the habit patterns of our lives—so any loss of upper weight carriage can easily be passed from one vertical position to another. *People who don't exercise regularly are especially vulnerable to a downshift of weight.*

When that downward tendency becomes a unconscious habit, the midsection bears the extra weight of upper body pressure and begins to fill out. Then the stomach, having no place to go (and probably too much food in it), protrudes, putting increased strain on the lower stomach muscles, which give way under the burden and are unable to hold it up any more. That means that the hips, buttocks, and thighs become the final resting place for excess weight.

By this time, the weight placement is way off balance, and the entire body is so far out of alignment that you've got anatomical and visceral problems. You're also stuck with a fat stomach that you can't hold in and large hips that look just as bad.

Unless you first learn to change your patterns and reset your body to its properly aligned style of uplifted carriage, no amount of exercising you do is going to make much difference, and it will probably make you tired, bored, uncomfortable, and discouraged.

Correct body posture is one that would allow a line to be drawn through the center of the three main bulks of body weight—head, chest and pelvis. With this invisible axis your body should be able to maintain internal–external balance and symmetry with an equalization of bone-and-muscle force and visceral activity. Body alignment means that everything is in its proper place doing what it is supposed to do.

When you unconsciously give in to a downshifted weight carriage and develop a disproportionate stomach and hips, your body is obviously out of alignment; its parts are out of place and are therefore not doing what they're supposed to do.

How, then, can exercise really be expected to reduce those parts if they're outside the very lines of movement that would reduce them? That's the frustration you face when you work yourself up to a lather doing spot exercises for stomach and hips without any visible progress. *Exercise, to be effective in reducing any one area, must be a line of movement through the body using all parts aligned together in a type of team effort.* Otherwise, you're wasting your time.

Even though corrective exercise is more effective in changing the body silhouette than changes in diet are, since too much food in the stomach definitely contributes to a fat stomach it's a good idea to reexamine your eating habits at the same time you decide to change your body shape.

Appetite is a sensation based on the previous experience of eating foods that taste good, and the memory of that experience is a pleasant one. Hunger is the desire to eat based on the need felt by the body when it has not had food for some time. Ideally, you combine the meaning of the two words in the process of satisfying eating desires. Unfortunately, many of us have an inclination to oversatisfy.

For weight control you need to determine the right balance of energy intake (food) and energy output (physical activity). When the calories consumed in food equal those used to meet your body's needs, your weight will remain about the same. When you eat more than this amount you will put on fat unless physical activity is increased proportionately.

It's possible to have fairly straight posture and still have a large stomach; it's possible to have a large stomach with small hips. That just means you're not quite as misproportionate as someone who's totally out of shape. But the prescription is the same for all—correcting the body carriage and exercising to put everything back in place, where it belongs, and then keeping it there. If you've been exercising and still have a large stomach, you haven't been doing the right kind of exercise.

That's why this book is called *The Tummy Trimmer Primer*, because the only way you're going to get rid of that stomach is to go back to basics, back to a "primer." You need to start over again, getting rid of all the bad body habits you've picked up and all the complicated, useless advice you've had on how to get rid of what you've accumulated.

The best way to begin the tummy trimming process is to learn the following basic exercise lesson.

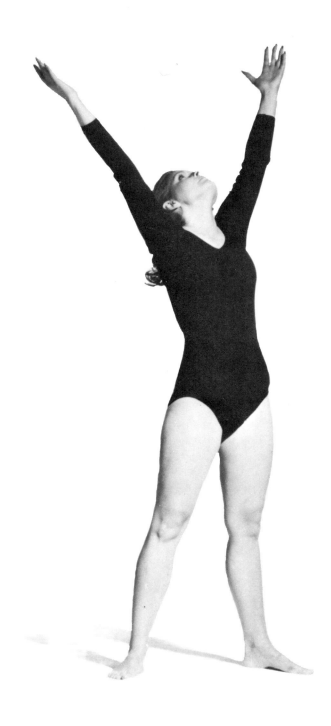

UPWARD AND OUTWARD

When you lift the rib cage slightly you create an extra inch of height through the torso at the waistline. Exercising in that position will pull your stomach in and up. Continued practice of exercises in this way will not only flatten the stomach and redevelop the strength to keep it flat but will also eliminate the excess weight in the hips and buttocks. Any exercise that pulls away from a large area will make it smaller.

To apply this basic principle, you use *stretch exercise*. Stretch exercise is a process of cooperative stretching and relaxing, stretching away from the body until weight becomes evenly distributed and muscles reach their maximum flexible strength. Other exercise styles concentrate on stationary and locomotor development of the body as it is, instead of correcting, positioning, and proportioning.

The style of stretching exercise is always upward and outward, emphasizing the lifting of your upper body so that the pressure is off the lower body. Exercising in an upward direction lengthens the vertical line through the center of your body and therefore makes the horizontal line through the middle more narrow.

This is an exercise system in which all areas of the body work together in natural, primary-movement directions, getting rid of large stomachs and hips in the process, as well as any other disproportionate areas. Do the exercises slowly so you can be aware of the subtleties in them that are so important for developing inner strength and control.

When your whole body works cooperatively in exercise movement the weight load of heavy areas is lightened because it is more evenly distributed during the action. As a result, you don't experience the usual exercise fatigue, because no one body part is forced to work harder to compensate for a part that's not being used. After all, the purpose of exercise is to reduce, reinforce, and strengthen, not exhaust.

These exercises do not call for great expenditures of energy, but they'll burn off calories at least as well as any other exercise does. After doing them you'll have more energy and feel better than you did before. They're simple to do, and they feel good, because your body moves without any body strain.

2

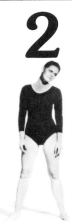

Preparing Your Body for Trimming

The stretch exercises in this book have been carefully chosen and arranged sequentially for best results. Don't do an exercise, or a set of them, out of context. Your body won't be properly prepared for each exercise and your results won't be as great.

If you wish to begin slowly, do only the warm-up unit on the first day. Then, add one more exercise each day, until you are doing the entire program every day.

When learned as a complete routine, with each exercise done slowly, four times, both sides equally, the whole program can be done in just about ten minutes. It shouldn't be hard to find ten minutes every day if you really want to have a flat tummy and narrow hips. Exercise is as natural a body function as eating and sleeping are. Everyone can find time to do this program.

Morning, before dressing, is the ideal time to exercise. The chances of sustaining the value of the exercises throughout the day are better when they are physically programmed into you the first thing in the morning. What's more, you'll find that the body stimulation is as good for you mentally and physically as a proper breakfast.

CHECK YOUR BODY FOR RELAXATION

If you have extra time in the morning I'd suggest you check your state of relaxation after you get out of bed. Occupational preoccupation that produces physical and mental tension carries over into sleep and sleeping positions. The retention of the subconscious mind-body is more powerful than you realize.

What does relaxation have to do with your tummy? When your stomach protrudes there is constant tension in the small of your back. Relaxing those tense back muscles allows the spine to straighten and draw in the abdomen. This checkpointing will give you a little edge on your morning exercising if you have the time to do it.

Presuming your floor is warm, lie on your back with ankles propped on the edge of a chair. (If the floor is cold you can do this lying flat in bed with comparable foot elevation.) When your body is relaxed, your feet will automatically fall apart; if not, they will remain pointed at the ceiling, parallel to each other. Let yourself go and unlock your body tension, and you will see your feet separate from each other and fall open to the sides. Then you are in a relaxed position.

POSITIONING YOUR BODY FOR EXERCISE

Since an uplifted position is the key to your tummy trimming success, the first thing to do before exercising every morning is to position your body accordingly. This preparation is important. With it you put your upper body in the position it should be in to do the very exercises that will give it the strength to hold that position. It's the first step in lifting the rib cage slightly to create that extra inch of height through the torso at the waistline. Exercising in that position is the action that will pull the stomach in and up.

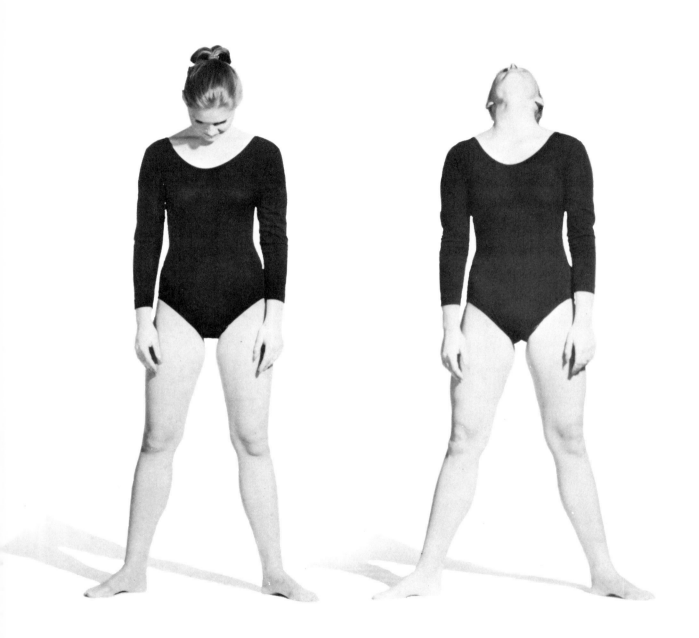

Stand naturally and bend your head forward as close to the chest as possible. Inhale slowly, and raise head to highest point as you lift rib cage. Exhale slowly, and move head backward as you maintain your uplift. Repeat three more times, inhaling deeply and striving for maximum height each time your head moves from front to back. In the

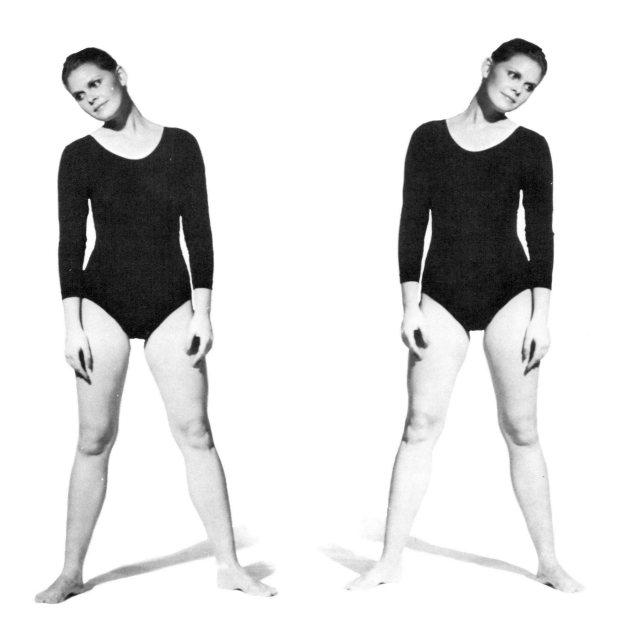

same uplift position, also move your head from side to side four times so you can be sure you've got the feeling of a raised chest all the way around your body. Because you are doing this very slowly, inhaling as you raise your head to the highest point possible, you should be able to reach extra height with the side to side head movement.

LIFT YOUR BODY—AND YOUR PRIDE

A sagging body implies a loss of physical pride. Positioning your body for exercise by lifting the rib cage should also set an emotional tone—pride. People who have tummy-hip problems suffer from a lack of confidence in their physical appearance, and therefore are handicapped by their own self-consciousness.

The commercial approach to exercise does not usually give people a sense of pride in what they are, but rather a feeling of guilt for what they aren't. According to such an approach there's always a perfect figure out there some place that you're supposed to have. The "perfect figure" that is commercially drawn is not the one to strive for: The perfect figure is your own when it is developed in natural proportion to your bone structure and body personality.

So, as you lift your body upward, lift your ego at the same time. Regardless of how big your stomach and hips are at this point, let your body wear a little pride, and any figure exaggerations will be less obvious. That alone should give you a little added motivation in your campaign against the bulge.

The position setting movements just described also loosen and stimulate your neck and upper spine for the body warm-up to follow. Tension in the neck and upper spine during exercise limits progress. Exercise will relieve your body of tension, but you get more out of your exercise and it's better for your body if you can get rid of some tension beforehand.

Since we are cerebral creatures it is more logical to begin movement sessions with heads—rather than feet, as so many unthinking exercise styles do. If you hear a lot of clearing or crackling noise in your head don't be frightened; it's just your sinus network trying to clear itself.

YOUR BRAIN MATTERS, TOO

One of the reasons people get so bored and give up on exercise programs is that they're doing something that doesn't involve their brain. To be able to sustain an interest in physical exercise your mind must be involved. Instead of feeling guilty that you haven't been able to stick with exercise, you should feel proud that you've got a brain good enough to rebel against movement that is meaningless to you.

That's why recreational exercise is usually the best individual all-purpose exercise there is. You swim, play tennis, handball, or golf because you enjoy it physically and mentally; your brain, the most important part of you, is not left out of the action.

But there's a lot of meaningless, treadmill type of exercise that people impose on themselves because they equate exercise with negative discipline—something you have to punish your body with. That's the way you were taught in school. "Forget your gym suit today? Ten laps around the track after school. Couldn't climb the ropes? Do twenty-five sit-ups." If you are interested in and enjoy jogging or sit-ups, do them; if not, you don't have to. Find something else that you like to do. There are many ways to exercise for good health.

3

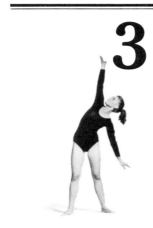

Warm-up Exercises

Most exercise forms use the flexor muscles more than the tensor muscles. Flexor muscles are muscles which bend; tensor muscles are muscles that stretch parts. Flexor muscles can do great things, but they can't smooth out the figure as well as tensor muscles. Stretch exercise is movement that is going up, out, and away from the body and therefore involves tensor muscle use. So, you want to be sure your individual stance is such that it can best handle this action—in direct proportion to your size.

For instance, if you are a tall person, place your feet far enough apart so that every movement you do will be comfortable. If you are a short person, your stance will not be quite as wide. When you exercise in a position out of keeping with your size, you distort your body and add to your problems. You will feel better when your movement proportions are complementary to your body type.

Everyone has a natural physical balance point that's determined by individual bone span, and it's necessary to apply it to exercise so that body leverage is neither inhibited nor pushed beyond its limit of strength. It's also more emotionally satisfying to exercise in relation to your size.

WARMING UP

Just as athletes, dancers, and even machines must be warmed up before full performance, so must you warm up your body before each exercise session. It's an easy procedure of gentle, gradual movement that stimulates the muscles and gets the body started.

Warm-up starts simply and builds on itself—from light movement to heavier movement. It's an overture, introducing your body to what's coming in the main exercises. Within this overture is a progression of movement; even though it's done slowly in respect to cold muscles, the warm-up exercises accomplish total muscle stimulation in a short time. Exercise warm-up is a means of mobilizing your body forces—organic and muscular—for better coordination.

Four warm-up exercises follow. You begin lightly with the first two, work up to the third, and return to the mood of the beginning as you do the fourth. This rhythm repeats itself throughout the entire exercise routine, taking on expanded movement patterns within its rhythm, tapering down at the end for best energy usage and body care.

Warm-Up #1

Standing in your uplifted posture, with feet comfortably apart, weight evenly distributed, slowly push your hands out to the side as if you were pushing out the walls. As you push your hands out look down at the floor.

As soon as you push your hands out to their farthest point, reverse suddenly and pull them in, and as you pull them in look up to the ceiling so that the torso will contract enough to gently stimulate the muscle control in the stomach.

Pretend you are pulling in the walls you just pushed out so that you can be sure of a reaction in the stomach, but not with such arm-muscle

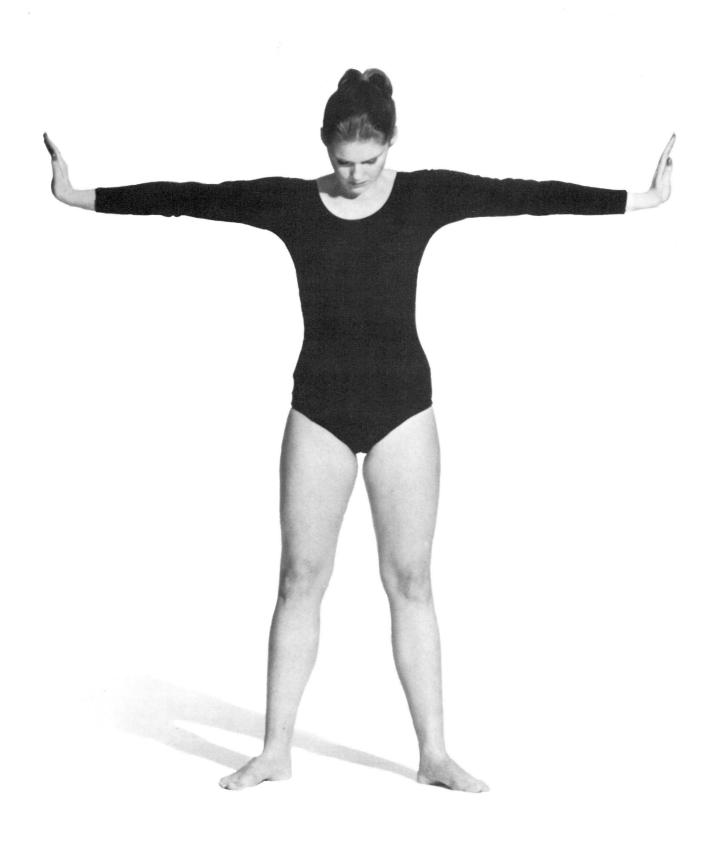

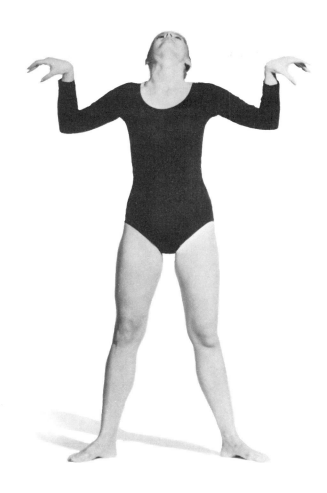

domination that it negates the fact that this is only a gentle body warm-up for the benefit of the stomach.

As you push the arms out you exhale; as you pull them in you inhale. The process of breathing with the exercises should become automatic—always exhaling as you go out from the body and inhaling as you lift and return.

It is possible that you might push out to such limits that you will quiver through the shoulders, arms and hands. Such zealousness in exercise is admirable, but not necessary here, because the point of this arm stretch is to allow the stomach muscles to automatically begin to tighten toward the spine.

After you have become more familiar with your individual energy spurts you can give as much to these movements as you want, as long as you don't start hunching in the shoulders, tightening up and forgetting the basic body uplift.

EXERCISE AND ENERGY

Energy is the capacity of the body to be active. Everyone's energy level differs, but in general, a noticeable lack of energy, shallow breathing, and general listlessness are signals that you need exercise. If you heed those signals and move your body around a bit you will generate more energy to do more things with greater zest.

Animals instinctively respond to such signals by moving their bodies; people do not, because they have gotten the idea that exercise is a separate physical endeavor to undertake when they have extra time. Watch a dog or a cat sometimes and notice that it stretches at waking and moves its body after periods of inactivity.

Sedentary living is very destructive. Not only do muscles atrophy if they're not used, but visceral activity like digestion requires more energy than just walking around. Exercise develops strength. *The stronger the body, the more energy it has and the more it will do for you; the weaker the body, the more it saps your energy and the more it demands from you.*

There's a reason for deep inhalation in exercise. It's been proved that the best exercises for basic human fitness are those that bring in the most oxygen to all areas of the body where food is stored so that the two can combine to produce energy when it is required.

Some examples of exercise forms that do exactly that are running, swimming, cycling, walking, handball, basketball, and squash. This type of exercise is called *aerobic.*

In all of the tummy trimmer exercises you're using the aerobic principle with your inhalation-exhalation patterns. If you want to go on from *The Tummy Trimmer Primer* to additional exercise that gives you more energy and enjoyment you might take up one of the aerobic sports, since they are also forms of pleasure exercise. They won't dramatically improve your figure, but they certainly will improve your health.

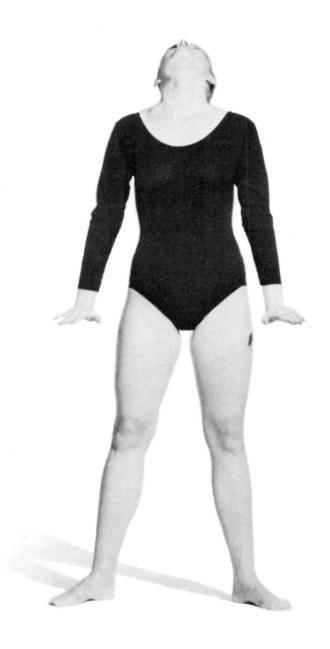

Warm-Up #2

    Push your hands down to the floor as you look up to the ceiling. This will continue the subtle torso contraction with a little more tightening of the stomach muscles. Notice that this is a palm push similar to the first warm-up exercise, and not a finger tip reach. That's done so that the inner arm muscles are stretched and therefore included in the warm-up. Every little bit of inner arm muscle usage is insurance against upper arm flab in the future.

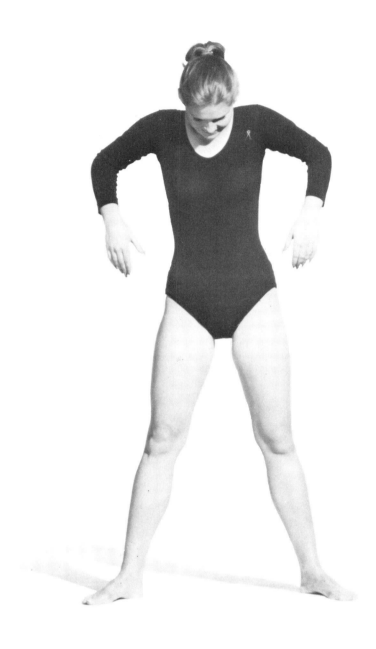

As soon as you push your hands as far toward the floor as possible, reverse suddenly, pull them up with relaxed fingers, and look down at the floor so that the torso will contract and pull your stomach in tighter toward the spine.

Keep your legs locked at the knees as you pull up, so that your rib cage will rise with the movement instead of caving in. You want your rib cage to develop dominant strength over your lower torso so that it can stay out of that area and stop crowding it with the extra pressure that makes the stomach protrude.

By keeping the legs locked and forcing the rib cage to rise with the movement instead of letting it cave in, you get a fully expanded inhalation in the chest. The most healthful exercises for the chest happen to be those that require full, complete and forcible expansion of its bony cage.

Why expand and develop the chest when your concern is with your stomach and hips? Because you can't begin to coax that stomach up and back into place if your rib cage isn't able to lift it. And if your stomach is very big and heavy, your upper body might have an even harder job. So you have to develop the chest.

The limits of your body expansion and development are only as great as your individual structure and capacity. Any visible expansion of a chest cavity will be in reasonable proportion to your size. After expansion reaches its limits, further exercise will only serve to strengthen and maintain it.

There are obvious, more attractive advantages to developing your chest, whether you are male or female. Well-developed chest muscles also give you a greater capacity for breathing, and for lifting the excess weight that has been pulling you down.

Warm-up #2 also encourages a lovely, long neck, but its most practical side effect is the accentuation of straight posture. The farther you can pull your shoulders down *behind* your body (with the force of your hand push) instead of parallel to it, the better your posture.

It is far better to do exercises that will develop natural good posture than to draw in your breath and throw your shoulders back when you try to be ultra straight. Every time you respond to your own straighten-up command you tense up, and then retreat to your habitual slouch for relief from the tension of tightening.

TENSION—ENEMY TO YOUR SHAPE

We've all made postural adaptations to our professions and individual lives, and most of these adaptations are not in good alignment with proper body carriage. So we've got to rely on exercise to keep putting us back in place. Otherwise, we slip into that weight shift that emphasizes our disproportions, and we waste energy and suffer from fatigue that pulls us down.

Occupations that employ small movements of the eyes and hands and that require many small decisions and judgments and much continuous attention can make our bodies tense. Sitting at a desk or sewing table, a typewriter or microscope, for instance, requires attentive tension—a readiness to move without using major movements. Tension results in fatigue. Fatigue combined with worry, anxiety, and pressure produces emotion that will manifest itself in a particular posture. Emotion always finds its expression in body position and then in body movement.

See how easy it is to get out of synch? That general responsibility of holding everything up is greater than you thought. As you do these warm-up exercises with wide-open ease, enjoy the immediate relief from tension.

Warm-Up #3

Clasp your hands behind your back, bend forward from the waist, and raise your arms as high as they'll go. Return to starting position and contract your torso with bent legs as if someone had suddenly grabbed your waist from behind. The stomach is pulled in tightly to the backbone as shoulders pull forward.

The contraction in the torso, which happens automatically in this movement, should become quite obvious to you now. If it doesn't, do

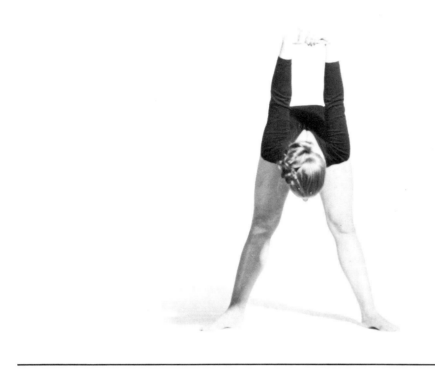

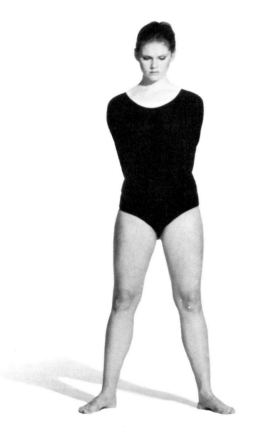

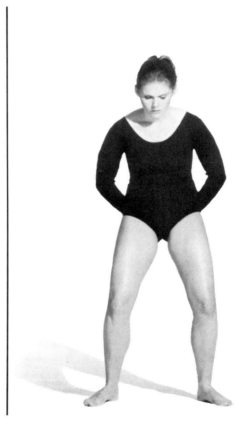

the movement again, being extra conscious of your lower stomach muscles by forcing some feeling into them. This third warm-up exercise is the climax of the introductory torso contractions, so it's important that you make mental contact with those inner muscle feelings.

Be sure to bring your body to a straight, upright position between each forward bend and contraction. It re-establishes a straight, high-held posture and gives form to the whole procedure.

Exercises should have form and style to them. That's what gives them purpose. Otherwise they are unintelligible and unmeaningful.

Think of form and style in exercise as synonymous with efficiency and grace. Each arm or leg movement should have a clear, confident direction to it as it relates to the torso action. There should be no random deviation from the line you wish to achieve, because that would weaken the action. A strong exercise is efficient and therefore graceful. A strong body with good muscle control is efficient and graceful; its exercise is done with form and style.

We learn and benefit most from what we learn with our physical senses. Mind and body constantly interact with each other if you let them. Be aware of what you're feeling in these warm-up exercises so that you can heighten those muscle feelings as you exercise further. There's a cumulative sensation of muscle control running through these exercises that is equal to your level of success.

Warm-Up #4

Reach to the ceiling with your left hand as you reach to the floor with your right hand, eyes to the floor. After reaching a maximum stretch point, reverse position and look down at the floor on the left side as your right hand reaches toward the ceiling. Reverse the arm positions again, but this time do the side stretch looking up at the ceiling. Reverse arms again and look up on the other side.

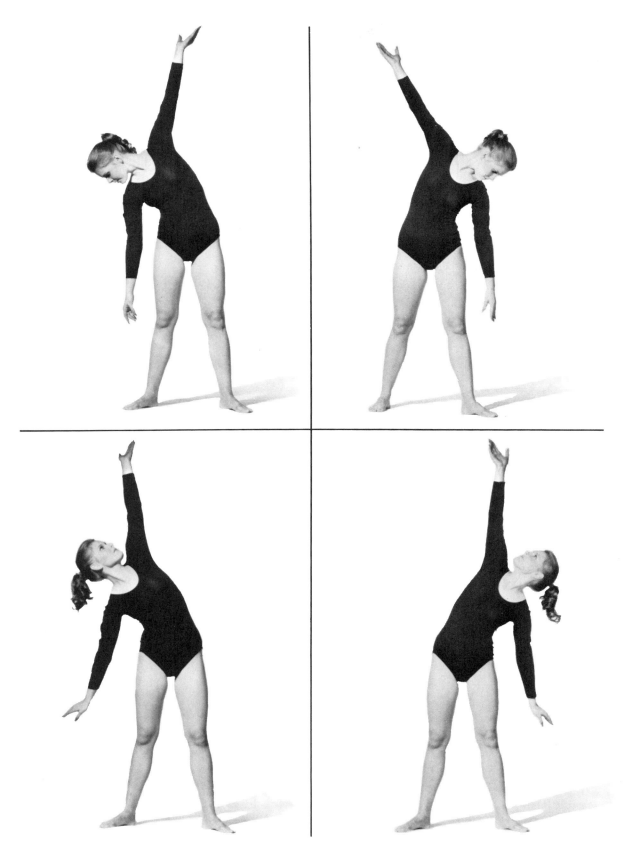

This fourth warm-up exercise is done for the purpose of gradually increasing your stomach muscle control and to warm up the sides that will be worked on later in other exercises. Each time the arms reverse position there is a sustaining contraction in the torso.

The reason you go through this looking first at the floor and then up is to give some of your smaller muscles a chance to be part of the whole effect. This happens with a shift of eye direction. The direction of the eye focus also gives more total direction to the movement, making it even more effective.

There is more to a good body warm-up than the motion would seem to suggest. In every warm-up there should be introductory, primary movement patterns established that relate to the style or the purpose of the exercise. Warm-up for football, running, and tennis varies according to the sport and whatever body proficiency you wish to highlight. In this book it's stomachs and hips, and the idea is to make them smaller.

In the warm-up series you've just done, the push—pull, tighten—release forces at work in the body as it stretches in different directions introduce valuable stomach muscle contractions, and they should not be missed.

A body contraction is muscle stimulation that pulls in and tightens, and it has great power to develop the control needed for a flat stomach after you have first lifted the rib cage and provided a place for the stomach to go. In the warm-up, the contractions happen naturally, without effort. As the exercises proceed you should be able to create your contractions with more conscious effort and give them even more power.

These exercises are not strenuous, but if you are just beginning an exercise program and wish to work up to it gradually, which is wise in any case, this is the point at which to stop the first day. It's a warm-up unit, but since it's also a general sampling of what's to come this set is a complete lesson in itself. Each day you may then add one more exercise in sequence until you have worked through the whole book and are then able to go through the entire routine daily from beginning to end.

If, for some reason, your regular exercise time is taken up by something else, you can always just do this quick warm-up series with the confidence that you are at least keeping up a basic body discipline. It's the same idea as having a nutritious snack if you have to miss a regular meal, or taking a brief cat nap if you're going to be robbed of your usual sleep.

Just be sure that you always do these exercises (and the ones to follow) in slow motion if you want to develop a harmonious internal—external muscle cooperation. That's what will give you a good total body personality and the image that's best for you.

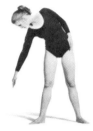

Standing Exercises

Now you're ready to move in more multi-dimensional stretch patterns. The first exercise in the next group slightly loosens the side-to-side torso action and begins the concentration of a stretch that will pull up the sides of your mid-section. This type of stretch also shifts body bulk into more proportionate balance, redistributing and getting rid of fatty deposits that have settled in the lower part of the body. Some people call the fatty deposits cellulite.

These exercises are meant to flow smoothly from one to the other without stopping, so that your body is able to experience a valuable continuity of form and style. When you learn all the exercises by memory you will be able to do that. But to help you learn the execution of the exercises and understand the nuances that will give special meaning to them they are separated in this book by supportive explanations.

Standing Exercise #1

Push your weight into your left hip to the left side as you reach out to the right with your right arm. Make a complete circle with the right arm going up, over to the other side, down across the front of your body

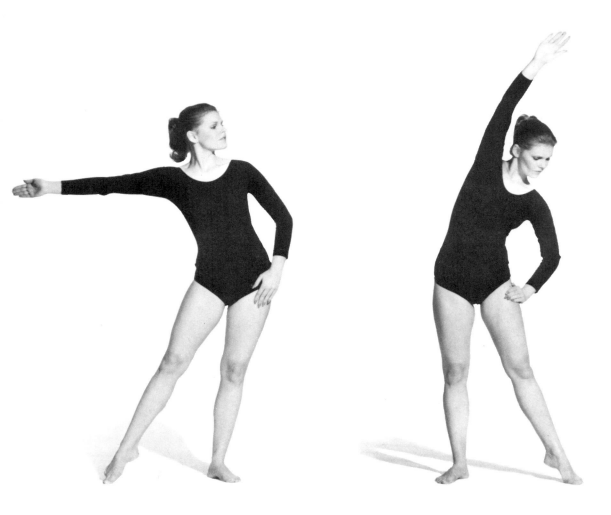

and back to its starting position. As your arm makes its unbroken circle, the weight of the body is shifted through the middle, into your right hip, back through the middle, and back to position. Be sure your arms and legs are directly to the side so there is no postural distortion; at the high point of the circle fully extend the arm reach (as in Picture 18). Do each side four times. If you are especially large in the hips complete each arm circle with an accent for extra pull.

You have within you the power to shape your body the way you want it. You only need to learn how to use that power and make it serve you. Presumably, what you want exercise to do for you is to proportion your body and make you feel good. But don't choose someone else's ideal body as your goal. It is more important to acquire control of the capabilities you already possess than to try to develop a body that doesn't become you or is not useful to your lifestyle. Therefore, in copying with your own body the exercises pictured, find yourself in the movements rather than trying to project yourself into the picture.

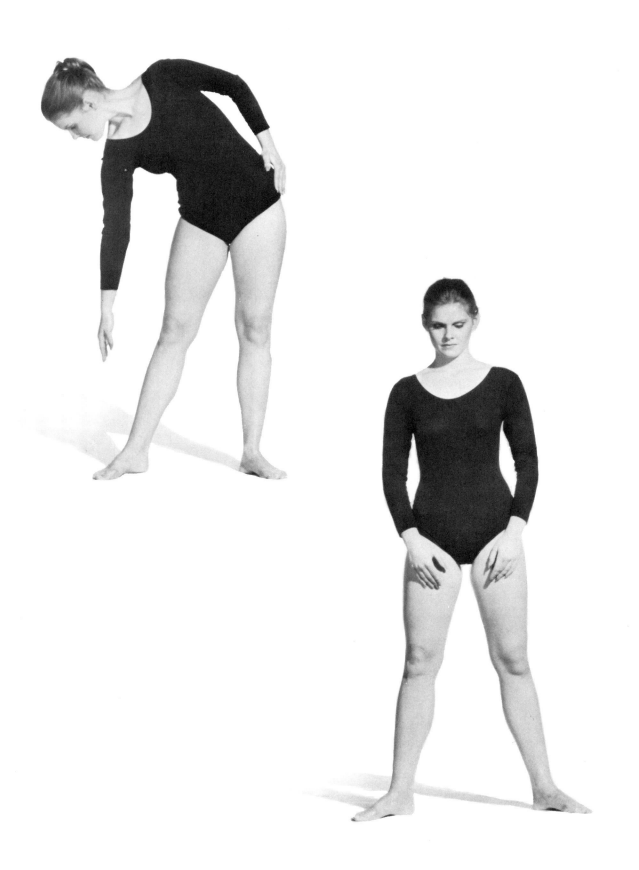

Standing Exercise #2

Bend to the right and reach toward the floor with your right hand. The hand must not be in front or back of the body as it reaches; it must be directly to the side so the body is kept in alignment. Reach and stretch with a gentle bounce four times and return to starting position, keeping your chest high and not letting it settle down into the lower torso. Repeat to the left.

In this series of movements, the stretch on the sides of the torso becomes more definite. Don't ever expect to reach the floor with your fingertips because the lower rib will meet the hip bone when you're bending directly to the side, as you should. But you can always work for more of a stretch on the outer line of the torso, and smooth things out a little more there.

Even though you do not have total physical control of your stomach yet, keep it mentally under control. Remember, there is a definite connection between mind and muscle, mind and motion.

With mind and muscle, mind and motion constantly interacting you've got the opportunity to control your body and have some power over it. If you have a protruding stomach and large hips your body has probably been controlling you.

Every body proficiency we acquire we learn by doing—walking, running, swimming, playing ball, etc. Anything we do with our bodies we learn by physically remembering how it feels to do it. All those body skills have a certain meaning to us and are useful in our daily lives for both practical and pleasurable purposes. Our heads are full of physical patterns we've put there by doing them.

Think about the exercises as you do them, and think about how they feel as you do them, so that interaction between mind and motion will make a useful physical-memory pattern. It will give you power over your own body now and in the future.

Standing Exercise #3

The last exercise of this side torso action is for the purpose of sustaining the side stretching and tightening you've just done and securing the feeling for your memory bank. Bend down and reach for the floor; reach directly to the side; reach for the ceiling; bring your arm down to its beginning. Repeat and alternate with the other side.

If you're not careful it's easy to revert to the "ONE –TWO–THREE–FOUR" loudly delivered cadence style of a school phys. ed. instructor, a memory that's guaranteed to drive out all individuality. Try not to let it happen, because it will stiffen you, and even though each position in this exercise is definite you want to be able to reach a maximum stretch at every point to help diminish your stomach and hips, rather than lock into a position that sets and accentuates what's already there.

But don't agonize if you do fall into the cadenced trap by mistake, because the next group of exercises will get you out of it.

If you're in the army or part of an exhibition drill team of some sort you've got to respond to cadenced exercise commands for the sake of group uniformity. The same thing is true if you are a part of a sports team and your body has to be in tune with a group pattern.

But if you are a man or woman who just wants to get rid of a protruding stomach and heavy hips you've got to allow your body to be an individual unit of expression and open it up to movement that goes beyond the limits of the cadence. Instead of trying to hold a beat and "keep time," phrase your movements.

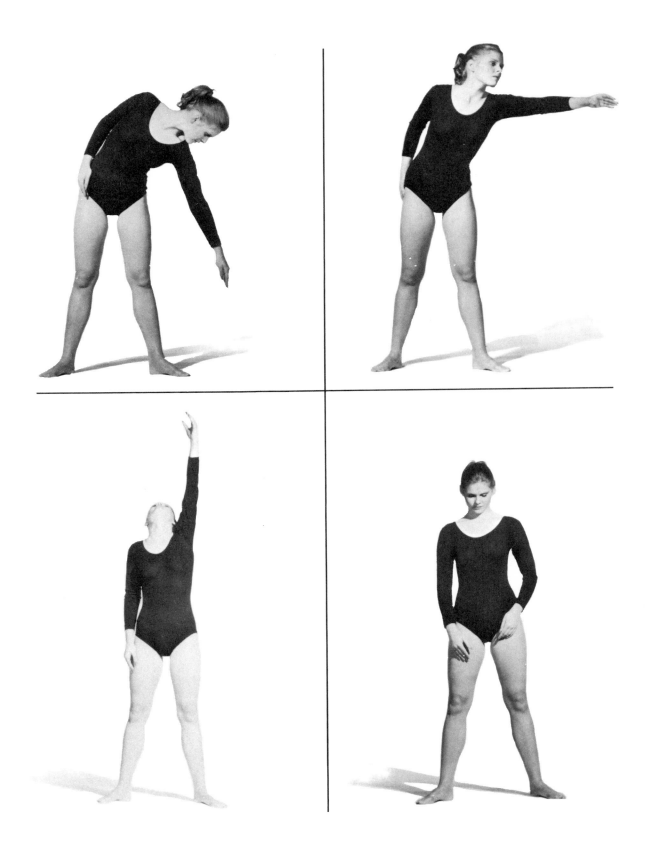

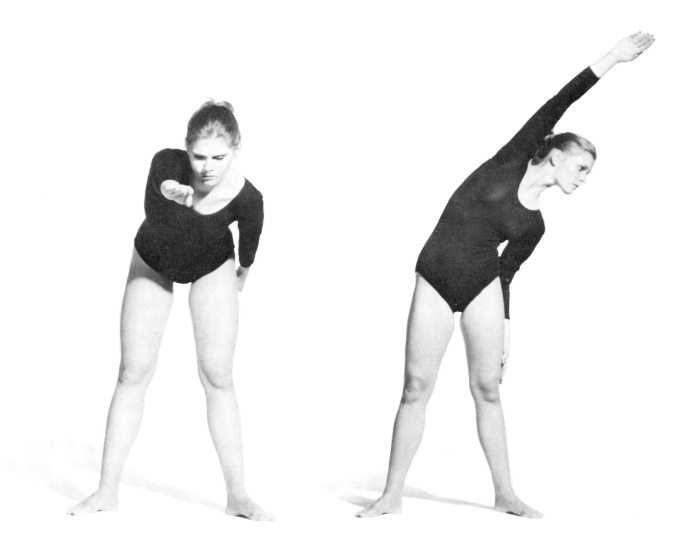

Standing Exercise #4

The torso has now been stretched up the sides and the stomach muscles have had some tightening and you're ready to make use of the extra height you've gained through the torso at the waistline. Now a circular motion is used to limber the torso so that it can develop a flexible strength. It's that flexible strength you need in the waistline to help you keep your stomach pulled up in the future. With this circular exercise you are practicing one more exercise that pulls away from the

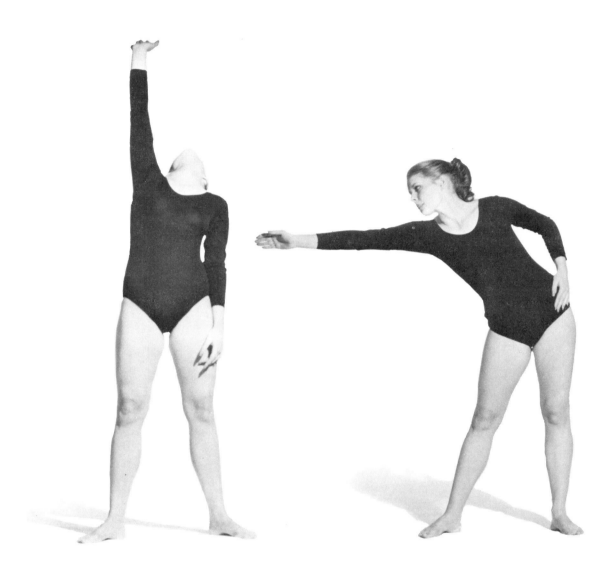

stomach to make it smaller, but you are also learning a waistline discipline that will be especially valuable in the future.

Bend and reach forward, then across your body to the left, back,
and to the right, striving the whole time to draw an imaginary circle on
each of the four walls in the room with your fingers as you make your
circle. Keep your eyes focused on your hands to prevent dizziness.
Should you feel insecure and off balance as you reach to the back, alter
your reach slightly so your arm is directed upward instead of back.
Repeat, reversing the direction of your circle.

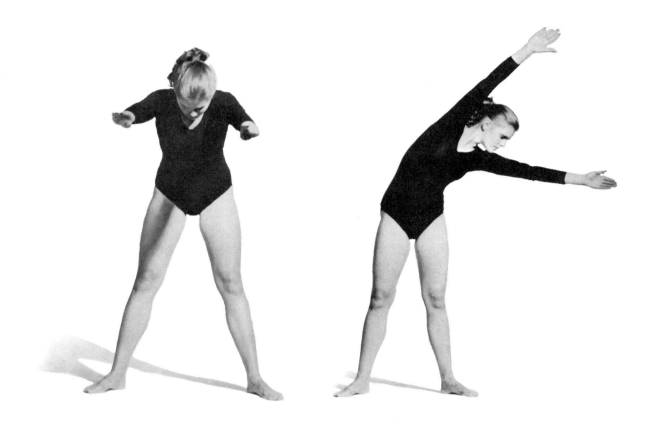

Don't ever be afraid to alter your exercise positions to conform to your own body. If you're tall and the exercise routine you're learning is being explained as if for the body of a short person, your stance must be wider than the one you see in front of you. If you're short and the pictures you are following are of someone very tall you must remember that your maximum reach is the point just before you lose your balance.

If you experience dizziness in a circle exercise, why should you jeopardize the benefit of the total exercise (and your own well-being) by forcing yourself to do it as it is when you can simply adjust it? If the exercise teacher can bring her head to her knees and you can't, don't punish yourself; you're getting just as much out of it by going to your limit.

Nothing is ever gained by straining your body. There is no reason to precisely duplicate the actions of another person in exercise. You've got to have enough respect for your own body to allow it to be what it is and develop as best it can according to your own body style. You can easily be receptive to your own body limits and capabilities and match them to the concepts and directions of the exercise. In that way you'll never need to fear injury nor will you think you're underachieving, because you will know your own body and have confidence in it.

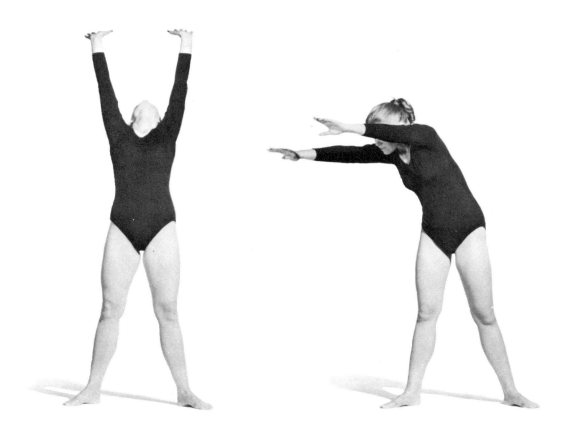

Standing Exercise #5

Here's your chance to really let go. After all, exercise should be as pleasant an experience as eating—which is why recreational exercise is so satisfying. So put yourself into this one with enthusiasm. It's big, and has a lyric quality to it; and, if you've not yet discovered the pleasure of exercising to music, by all means try it.

This is the tightening and sustaining exercise for the circular movement just done. You do it the same way you just did the single-arm circle but with two arms instead of one. With the one-arm circle you established your body balance; with the double-arm circle you exercise your central power of control.

This exercise, along with Standing Exercise #4, will help you understand how to control your own body. Any time you have an exercise that you do with a single arm or a legs-together position and then repeat it with double arms or legs apart you are mastering control of your midsection. Note it, and remember the feeling so you can work with it.

You may have tried other exercises that were supposed to be good for the waistline only to become discouraged by fatigue and your lack of success. There are sit-ups, elaborate body twists, windmills, leg lifts, and many others. Every one of those exercises has its own muscle-toning value, but if you study them closely you should be able to see that they do not really make the waistline smaller.

The only way you can have a smaller waistline is to separate your upper body from your lower body so that you can actually create an indented shape. Twisting, bending, sitting up, or lifting your legs will not do it. When the waistline is subjected to that type of movement there is no place for the extra inches to go, so they remain at the waistline. But if the upper and lower torso are pulled apart, the waistline becomes narrower just by its altered posture.

When you do these stretch exercises, pulling excess flesh up and away from your waistline, you are proportioning your body as you work the fat off. You're actually using your waistline as an instrument to shift the stomach and hip excess. Your waist must be identifiably between the upper and lower body instead of in the middle of the mass, so that it can act as a flexible link and become strong by its action.

Every time people rise out of their sedentary lives to do something about their bulging bodies they start trying to bend over and touch their toes every morning. They huff and puff away without realizing what they're really doing to themselves.

There are many people who will never be able to do that exercise as it was taught them, because of their particular body structure. To bend over and touch your toes with considerable ease your bone structure must be the same proportion from waist to head as from waist to feet. Otherwise, you're straining your spine to do something it's not constructed to do. When you have a large stomach, touching your toes is impossible because your stomach acts as a barricade.

This next exercise changes the traditional position for toe-touching so that it can be done by any body and any shape, with more spinal

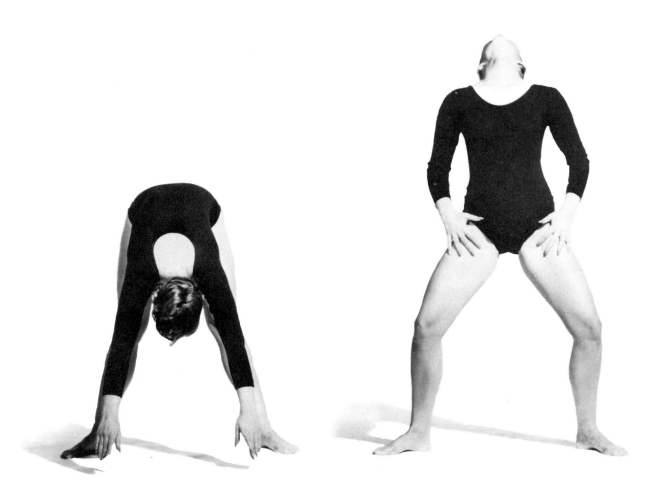

leverage, which means a reasonable amount of ease and no unnecessary strain, and you can expect success and benefit from it. As you reach forward, your stomach can easily be pulled toward your spine. Each time you go back the stomach pull toward the spine is tightened. There is also a pull up the backs of your legs and across your buttocks as you go forward that is effective in smoothing extra bulk.

Standing Exercise #6

Spread your feet instead of doing this exercise with them together, and reach for the floor in front of your feet rather than for your toes. Reach forward four times with straight legs and then bend back as far as comfortable and hold to a count of four, letting your legs bend slightly as you go back. Repeat forward and back four times.

When you are able to touch the floor in front of you with your fingertips, in Standing Exercise 6, try next to touch with flat hands, then elbows (some people are very long waisted and might be able to do so). Do not bend back any farther than is comfortable, or you will strain your back unnecessarily.

Any time you need to pick something up from the floor you might get into the habit of doing it with this exercise instead of bending down to the object. It's a good idea for people who think they never have time to exercise.

There are many ways you can integrate these exercises into your daily routine. The most elementary example is to stretch to maximum in all positions every morning when you wake. This feels very good and is good for you after the inactivity of a night's sleep, because it brings oxygen into your system. This oxygen helps stimulate your circulation and the movement will gently awaken your muscular system.

In the shower, stretch your stiff muscles under the warm water, bending down smoothly to pick up the soap while you're at it. When dressing, make the entire muscular network of your torso and limbs work together as you pull on socks or step into pants, rather than dressing with separated leg and arm motions that take more energy.

We've been considering three kinds of exercise interchangeably:

1. Corrective exercise to correct a deformity
2. Hygienic exercise for general good health
3. Mental exercise to control it all

It's all one force behind the concept of lifting, changing posture settings, and shifting weight masses, whether you do it within the discipline of an exercise period or as part of your other daily functions.

An exercise that pulls your stomach in and tightens it tends to make the stomach smaller and control it. An exercise that pulls up the buttocks and pulls weight off the hips tends to make those parts smaller. An exercise that moves a part in the direction it must go to be in its proper place has the power to correct that part.

Total body exercise that moves along muscular lines from toes to fingertips is exercise that does just that. That's why people who dance, swim, play tennis, or regularly indulge in similar activities have better looking figures than those who don't. Their bodies are in constant stretching movements that maintain their parts in proper placement and control.

Such movement is not limited to one or two dimensions, as some traditional stationary exercises are. The stretching is going on, open and unconstricted, from many directions and in many angles. If you want to accomplish the same thing, you have to do your total body exercises from many angles too.

Standing Exercise #7

Since you should be feeling some muscle control in the stomach at this point, the next exercise will go on to build more control from a different angle—back side to opposite front side. More stomach muscles are used in this exercise because of the cross pull that comes up the backs of the legs and across the buttocks.

Notice that the body does not twist in the torso, so that the natural stretch line, along which the stomach will move, will be kept open. Proportioning cannot take place if your body sections are not working in reciprocal motion.

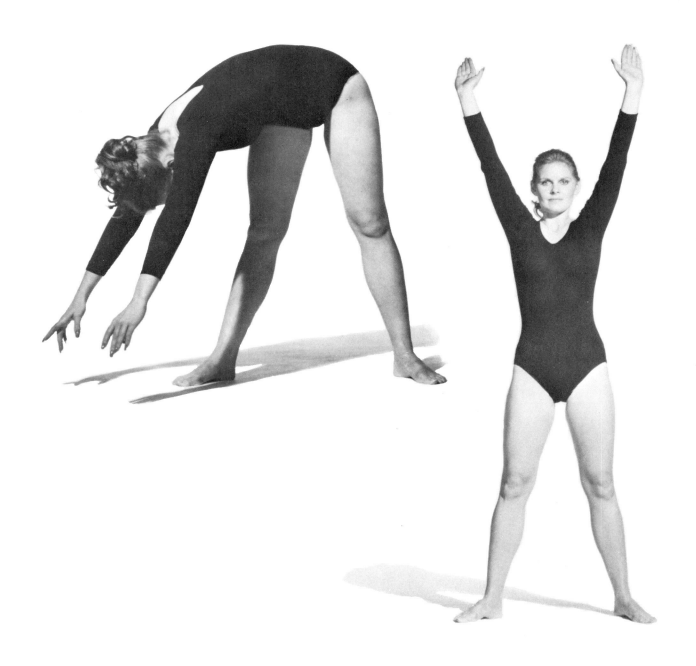

Stretch with both hands to one foot, stretch up, then stretch to the other foot. Your legs must be kept straight and your weight must be kept evenly distributed on each foot. It is important to maintain a maximum stretch throughout the whole exercise so that at no time is your body allowed to sag.

If the direction of your movement is to one side but you are instructed to keep your weight evenly distributed you must exercise almost as much mental control over movement as you do when you try to

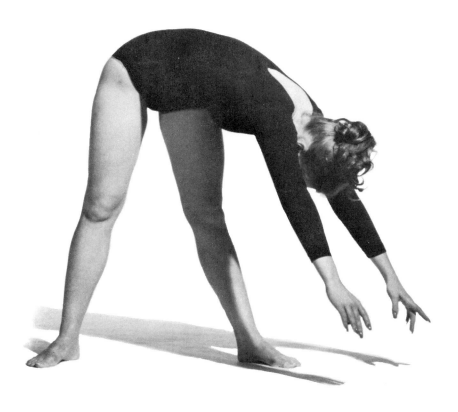

pat the top of your head with one hand and rub your stomach in a circular motion with the other hand.

You could more easily have done the last exercise by shifting your weight to each side, but then your stomach muscles wouldn't have gotten any strengthening benefit and you would have lost an opportunity to practice controlling your body. Mental muscle control over movement is an accomplishment.

Compare the exercise you just did with one you might have done in the past: twisting in the waist and reaching for your opposite foot as the other arm is thrust out in back. Your old way destroyed the natural movement line of the body by twisting in the waist, so even though it allowed you to keep your weight evenly distributed it didn't budge the stomach.

Simplicity is frequently the answer to a problem. When things become complicated and nothing works it's good to erase everything, return to a beginning, and start over. That's when you discover the basic concept, the single line, the essence and beauty of the thing you've been laboring with that your very complex mind has lost sight of.

There's a single line of thought and action to *The Tummy Trimmer Primer:* the uplifted body line that goes through the three main bulks of body weight—head, chest, pelvis—and that lets everything be properly in place doing what it's supposed to do in a balanced, proportioned way. That's the answer to the problem of the large stomach–hip area. It can't be more simple and obvious.

To see it, stand in front of a mirror and shape your body to that line. If you've been doing the exercises correctly up to this point you'll be able to feel that line as you see it. Never mind that you also see your bulging stomach. It will disappear as you exercise in that simple, unifying body line of direction.

The body assumes the style of the exercise it practices most, so if you're going after a particular image you want to be sure to exercise accordingly. Most of the exercises in this book are graceful and therefore flattering to the body line.

To achieve a lasting, smooth, graceful line from an exercise, the movement has to be done from within. You'll notice isometric principles involved in this next exercise, in the sense that you are building the muscle strength that will give you the power to hold in your stomach. It's an inner muscle development that will never show, but it will serve you well.

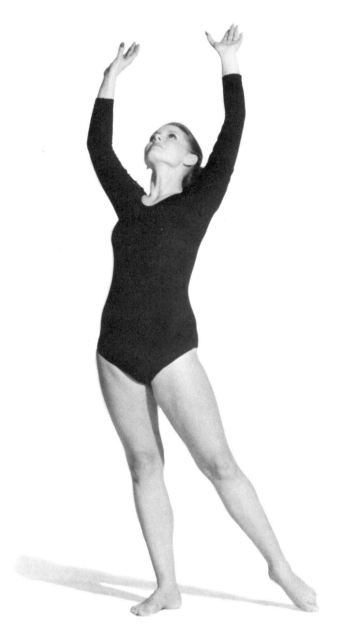

Standing Exercise #8

Push your weight forward into your left hip slowly, letting the result be an arched back with your arms and right leg trailing behind and giving the illusion of a smoothed-out body in front. For the sake of your lower back, do not strain. When you push to the point of balanced control pull back to position, making sure you use your inner stomach muscles to do so, as you continue to hold the whole body line up with your arms.

All the exercises in this book can be done by either men or women. They are basic stretch exercises that have their roots in dancers' exercise. Many of them resemble yoga movements. They are very effective for stomach control and body proportioning, regardless of age or sex.

Stretch exercises have become part of the conditioning programs of many college and professional track and football teams because they prevent hamstring pulls and other muscle injuries. Athletes use stretch exercises before their heavy body workouts to develop flexible muscle strength. They also use them after the workouts to draw the lactic acid out of their systems and cool their bodies down. Stretch exercises are very graceful because they are so efficient and natural.

What most people need from exercise is the flexibility, body strength, and endurance that comes from doing this type of movement. It's one of the best ways to stay in shape and prevent large stomachs and hips in the future.

5

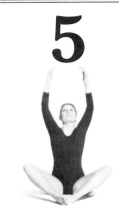

Sitting Exercises

Animals, moving through their lives in the exact structural position they were born in, only have to concern themselves with horizontals, the position we use in bed. We've got those daily skeletal adjustments to make between vertical and horizontal positions, keeping our bodies pleasant to look at and in good working order at the same time. Generally speaking, we do quite well because our ability to think and reason coordinates our physical and mental activity.

But it is mental activity that dominates us, and in our vertical positions we tend to lose what the animal retains—muscle instinct. Everything the animal does on its horizontal plane it does with power from its haunches; our power comes from our brains. So you see, it isn't totally your fault if you've lost control of your abdominals. We're all vulnerable to the mental dominance that ignores our muscle power.

When you forget your physical need to hold everything up in favor of your mental preoccupations, and the abdominal muscles are no longer able to engage in their reciprocal action with the diaphragm, the stomach—hip problem is compounded when you sit, especially if you don't exercise regularly.

In a sitting position, as in a standing position, there is the same necessity to change your posture patterns and reset your body to its properly aligned style of uplifted carriage. You might think you're sitting properly if your back is straight, but you're probably letting all your muscle control go, so that the weight is resting in your hips and buttocks. There it stays while the fat piles up even more in the stomach above it.

People who have large stomachs, hips, and buttocks habitually sit with their bodies incorrectly placed; they sit on their largest part and encourage continued growth of these body parts through incorrect weight placement.

You've got to learn to sit with your body weight held up instead of released, sitting away from your largest part instead of right on it, leaning slightly forward instead of back. This does not mean that when you sit you should be stiff as a soldier. It simply means that you shouldn't sit like a rag doll.

You should be able to get up from a sitting position as easily as you got down to it. If not, it means that when you sat down all the muscle control in your body was released. To get up again you have to re-mobilize the body forces needed to get you up. That takes extra energy away from other parts of the body.

There's a difference between relaxing your muscles and letting them go completely; you can relax a muscle or set of muscles and still keep them alert and ready for action. The key is posture control, being in alignment, and remaining aware of your stomach muscles, all of which can be developed with exercise.

The purpose of exercising while you sit is to make body maintenance—especially of your stomach and hips—a more naturally automatic process by strengthening the muscles used in proper sitting. This sets off a chain reaction that will give you far better proportions, more flattering body lines, and correct weight carriage.

If you stretch or do any other forms of sitting exercise before first checking your position, you may strain your back, and you will probably always have larger hips than necessary. *Keep your lower back from bearing all the weight so that the body is always able to move freely and without strain in its sitting position.*

To accomplish this, lift the weight from your hips through the whole torso and incline very slightly forward, a simple shifting of weight placement. That simple shifting of weight placement keeps the weight from settling. Teach your body this uplifted position for daily use but use it especially for sitting exercises.

A popular, but very ineffective sitting exercise is rolling from side to side on your buttocks and hips. It not only breaks heavy tissue down to flab, but the downward pressure created just increases size and creates more flab. The whole idea is to pull the weight away from the enlarged area so it can get smaller and tighter.

Another exercise that's over-rated is the sit-up. Few people have the necessary strength in the stomach-pelvic area to do sit-ups correctly, and if they are not done correctly they don't do much good. When you don't have adequate strength to take your torso up to a sit, you compensate by using your back muscles for the moving force, leaving your stomach muscles to get their strengthening second hand. As a result, your stomach muscles never develop a strength equal to their backside helpers.

The strain involved in doing a sit-up is fatiguing, discouraging, and physically unnecessary. There's nothing wrong with the exercise; it's just that it should be done to *maintain* torso strength, not to develop it.

People who like sit-ups and want to do them would be wise to do some isometric stomach muscle exercises first. A good one is to lie in bed and tighten your stomach and buttocks muscles so hard that your knees rise slightly, and then release. Repeat the tighten-release pattern three times. People, however, who don't like sit-ups and don't really want to do them don't have to.

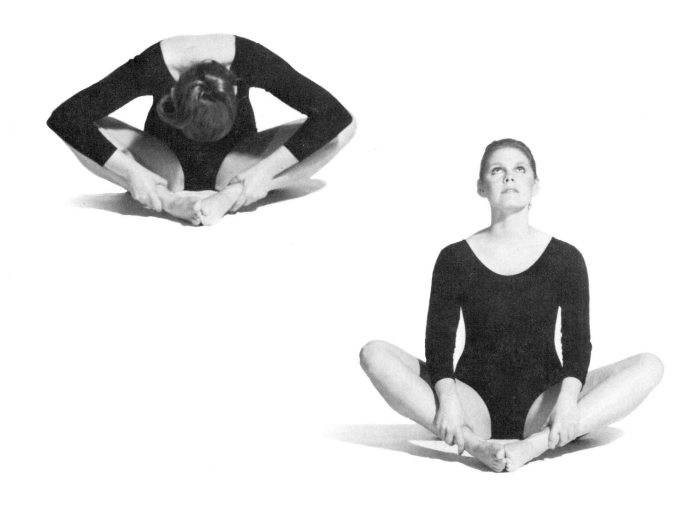

Sitting Exercise #1

Before you do the following sitting exercises, go back to the beginning of the book and do the head exercise for body positioning, just to be sure you set your body in that uplifted position. Even though this first sitting exercise goes forward toward the feet it must be going out and down from an uplifted position to create as much flexible space through the midsection as possible.

With soles of your feet together, hands holding your ankles, gently pull your head as close to your feet as possible. Repeat for a total of eight times. Without any conscious effort your stomach will be pulled toward the spine. At the same time, any extra bulk will be pulled up the back of the buttocks.

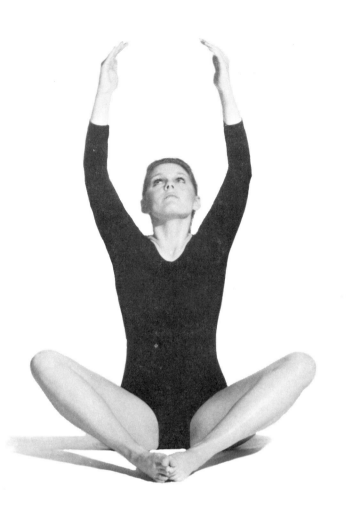

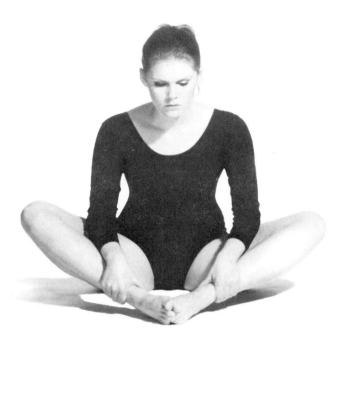

Whether or not your head actually reaches your feet is not as important as your effort. The exercise will benefit you regardless of your degree of limberness. In time, of course, a more limber body will develop naturally, but that is not the immediate goal. Your concern should be slow, smooth stretching that pulls the stomach in and up while it smooths the back line and straightens the spine, centering your body as it does so.

Pull up to a straight, high, sitting position that is inclined very slightly forward and hold it for two counts. The action is pull in, lift up, and hold. Raise your arms high to exaggerate the upper body lift and hold this position for two counts. Release, relax, exhale and repeat three times.

You'll find it difficult at first to hang on to the position with arms held high and, at the same time, maintain that straight spine, but do the best you can. The development of a stronger, straighter spine is worth the effort. Return hands to ankles, and pull forward with a straight back four times, chin leading slightly to pull out any neck kinks you might have gotten while you held your arms up.

Make sure you inhale as your arms rise and completely exhale when you release the position. It is natural to do so but I mention it so you will strive for maximum inhalation and exhalation. You might as well benefit your body in little bonus ways like bettering your circulation while you work on stomach and hips.

Centering describes the adjusting of symmetry that goes on in the body during any exercise that is done with contained movements in definite directions. When you stretch your head toward your feet with your hands placed equally on each ankle for support, your point of direction is between your feet so your movement is forced into an exact middle line.

Even the most aligned, most fit, and most nearly figure-perfect person has brief deviations from his base of control. Centering exercises provide a built-in process that is its own check-and-balance system. For example, if the spine is put into alignment down the middle of the back, the head can then be properly held atop the neck, and the shoulders will become squared.

Good muscle control is more easily achieved in a symmetrical body. If the stomach is to be put in its proper place and kept there, the supporting areas must also be put in their places. You wouldn't really want to have a flat stomach and narrow hips encased in an otherwise misshapen body anyway.

There are many aspects to the subject of exercise, so in your quest for a flat stomach and narrow hips you cannot be concerned only with those two body sections. Every once in a while you have to pause and get a perspective on the whole person who is employing that exercise for good health and a better figure. Consider the effects of some of the other factors involved so that you can integrate them into your movement. I've already mentioned breathing and your pattern of inhaling and exhaling with a movement in connection with previous exercises.

Breathing is a natural coordinating mechanism for all the body forces. There's a whole chain of muscles that take part in the breathing process, such as the deep lying abdominal and pelvis groups. When you exercise, you enter into a breathing pattern in which you can cleanse and refresh and stimulate your circulation to a greater extent if you work with the motion. If you exercise in the more shallow breathing rhythms of your daily routine, you don't get as much organic value.

The real foundation of good health is organic, but you can't separate the inner and the outer person, and you can't have good organic health without exercise that creates a deep, rhythmic breathing pattern.

Sitting Exercise #2

Leaning slightly forward, reach for the ceiling, one arm at a time, being conscious of teaching that uplifted-torso sitting position to the muscles along the sides of the body, and reaching a little higher each time you alternate. This works off the fat accumulation along the ribs; the more earnest the reach, the more fat removed. Repeat two times each side.

If you spread your legs and repeat the exercise you can get even more out of it. Note the side line in which the hips are flattened because of the exercise. Feel the heaviness being pulled out of the buttocks and hips, through the midsection and upper body, and off. Feel the delightful torso separation you're now able to accomplish, and retain it.

The practice of a set of movements like this tends to shape the parts accordingly. It should be very obvious that the entire stomach—hip area is becoming narrower.

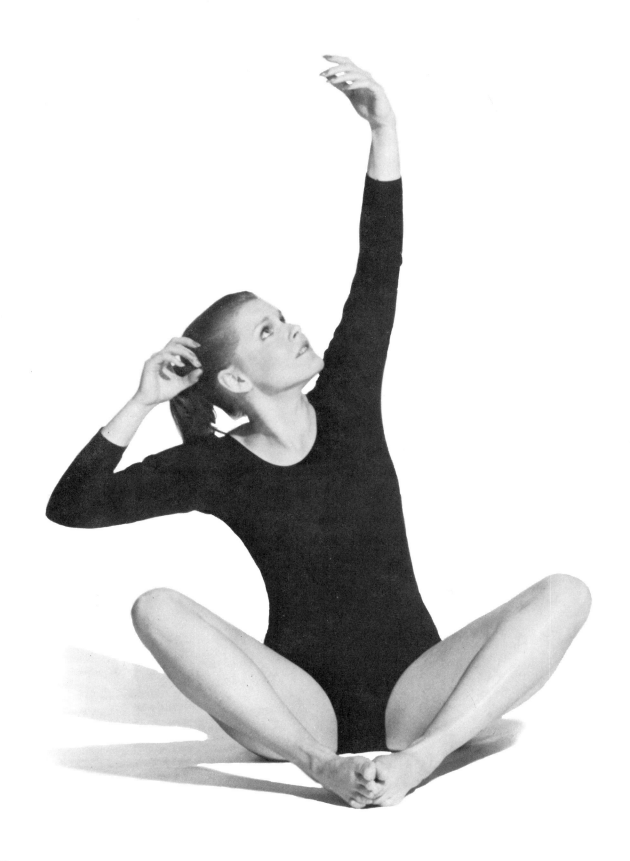

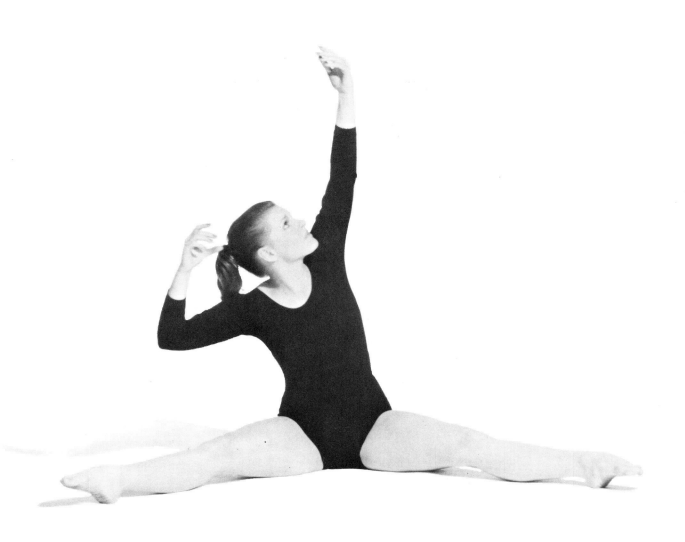

To look the way you want, you have to teach your body the way you want it to look and give it examples, doing exercises that actually put it in place so the muscle memory can take it from there.

Most of the exercises people have been taught to do for large areas are movements that accentuate them by flexing and featuring them. But the real progress is in the exercises that diminish, and draw away from those areas. The benefits of the exercises in this book that diminish the stomach are not obvious from the pictures because most of the action is going on inside. The pulling-away principle is easier to see in the hips.

It's the hips and buttocks that become the final repository for excess stomach weight, so it's illogical to resort to hip rolling thinking you're working if off. Haven't you ever noticed that people who sit the most on their largest mass grow larger? *Get off it and get rid of it.*

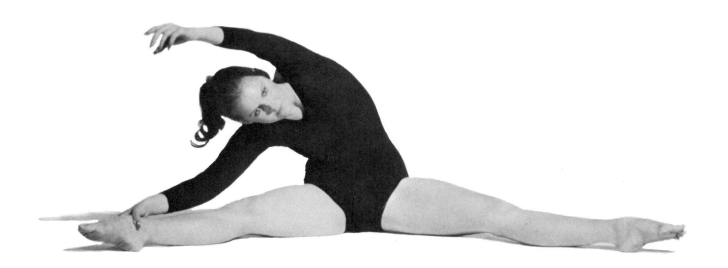

Sitting Exercise #3

The most powerful exercise for getting rid of excess bulk along the torso lines is this side to side stretch. It's an obvious example of the body sections working together for proportioning. You usually see it done with a twisted reach to the alternate foot, but the open stretch shown here is far more effective because it doesn't cut off the main body sections from each other and render them useless in partial motion.

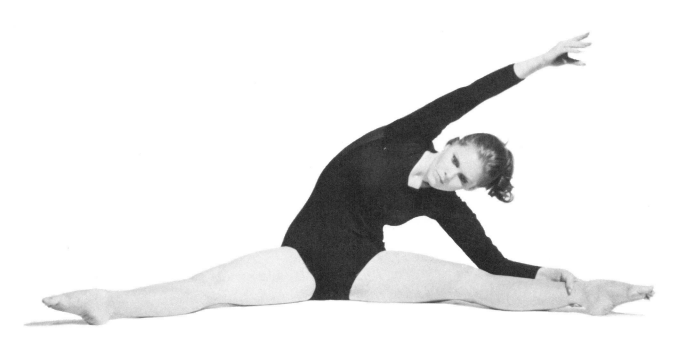

The more you do this the more limber you become, which means the more flab you are able to pull off and tighten in a flexible manner. When the excess has been worked out of the torso—hip area the movement will begin to pull fat away from the heavy thighs.

With your legs spread a comfortable distance apart, reach directly to the side as far as possible to a count of four. Do it slowly for maximum reach. If you are especially heavy in the hips do the exercise with palm turned upward for extra pulling power.

When you digest the information between the pictures and learn to do the actual exercises in this book so that you can go through them *every day consecutively* and without stopping, you'll realize that there's a definite structure and rhythm to them. Everything is done four times, each side equally either two or four times, in a general overall four—four time.

Within the general rhythm of the exercise plan you should also realize that each set of movements is followed by a counter set. It's one of those unwritten rules of good exercise which complements the tighten—release, stretch—relax, plus—minus, yin—yang theory or any other law of physical nature that applies.

Exercise should enhance the body, not distort it. Even the corrective exercise for large stomachs and hips must be done within a natural rhythmic structure. You cannot separate body sections and expect them to relate to the whole in a harmonious way. So don't lose sight of the whole even though this book is basically dedicated to the protruding parts.

Sitting Exercise #4

With your legs spread as far apart as is comfortable, pull your head toward the floor four times. You will probably not be able to get all the way down to the floor as in the second picture, but that is not important. What is important is what's happening as you do it. This is a maximum-benefit exercise in which the stomach is pulled tightly in toward the spine. The pull up the back of the buttocks is similar to the first sitting exercise. It's a saucer shaped, smoothing action, slightly concave in front and gently rounded in the back. That action is made even

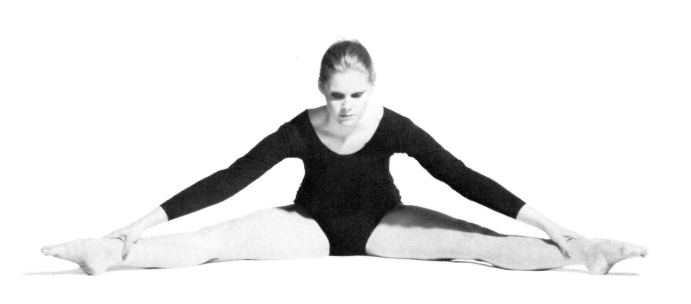

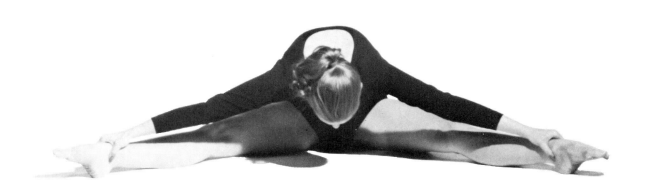

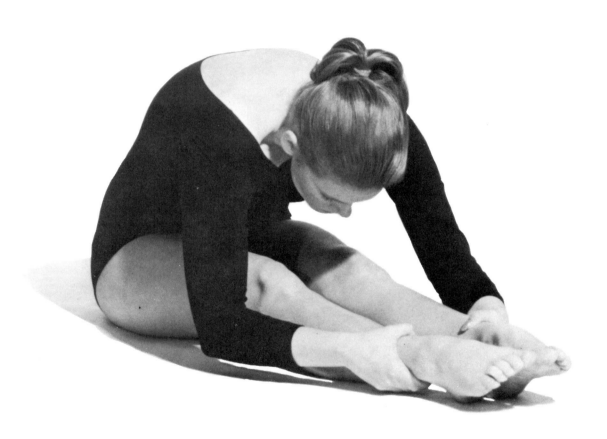

more definite when you do it with the legs together, as shown—an exercise you can repeat in the bathtub for extra benefit if you want to.

Because you are stretching forward with your legs in a straight position, you will notice a slight pull in the muscles of your inner thighs. If it bothers you, don't spread your legs so far apart until those muscles become more accustomed to it. Realize, however, that stretching those inner leg muscles will also control flabbiness in the upper legs.

Your knees may want to jump up slightly as you go forward, but force them to stay down. When you can control your knees, you'll know you have also developed some stomach control.

The limits of movement are determined by the structure of the body. That's what makes stretch exercise so good for so many people—men, women, children, and people with special problems like large stomachs. Stretching exercise is self-induced movement that reaches out from the body instead of movement imposed on the body. You will get out of it what you put into it and what you are meant to get from it, and it will be in keeping with your own body style and shape and that's a very valuable benefit.

Every person's body is different in size, shape, and the way it's put together. Each problem is different. An exercise that can be done easily by one person might give another person trouble. You must consider factors like short waist or long waist, leg lengths in relation to torso, and muscle tone. There are also many exercises done for figure development and control that should only be done by a body that's already in good shape.

So adjust the leg and arm spans of the exercises in this book to your own points of comfort so that each exercise becomes yours. Don't be discouraged by the fact that the picture shows more than you can do. Learn how to do the exercise, understand the point of it, and do it in confidence in harmony with the structure of your own body.

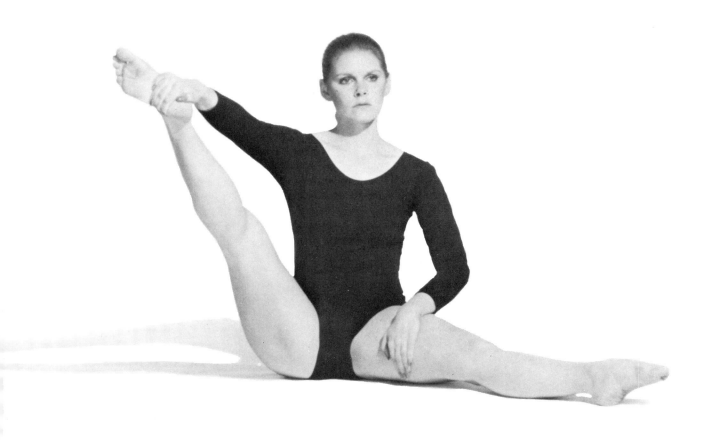

Sitting Exercise #5

This exercise shows the rewards you'll reap after you learn, and begin to do regularly, the exercises in this book. Starting with a single leg, extend it to the side as shown, tightening the stomach muscles in the process. Then extend both legs at the same time and hold. It takes total control of your stomach muscles to be able to do it without rolling backward, but it represents mastery over the undisciplined stomach you

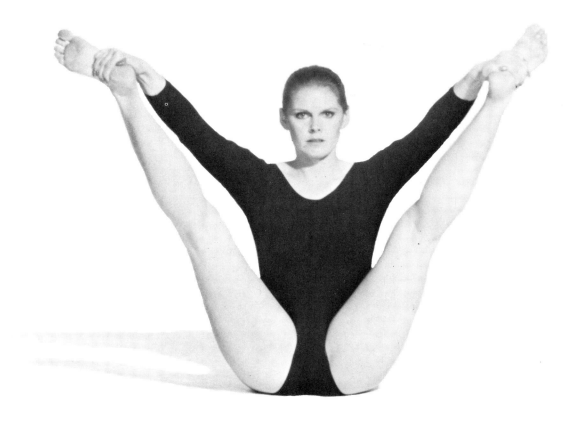

started this book with. Repeat four times with each leg and four times with both legs.

In order to hold the posture of this exercise, the stomach muscles must tighten involuntarily so that the leg can extend and stretch. This muscle tone cooperation develops strong balance throughout the body and helps in keeping the body held high.

Who would think that an exercise featuring the legs would be so good for the stomach—hip area? But the relationship of the stomach muscles to the leg muscles in this exercise is very important. It looks as if only the leg muscles are in use, but there is an invisible force at work that involves the whole body in a controlled position.

I've taken you through an exercise routine for your stomach and hips that began standing and ended sitting, working up to a point of maximum exertion and then tapering down. You should feel good. You will feel even better if you don't let everything go when you stand up.

Keep your body uplifted and try to sustain all the feelings of shifted weight and muscle control as far into the day as you can. Each day those feelings should last longer and longer until you get to the point where they are with you all the time. When you've reduced the size of your tummy and hips you will also have developed the strength to keep them flat, especially if you practice some kind of regular exercise.

The movements you've done make a fine basic daily exercise plan if you wish to stay with them. They keep the rest of the body trim, too.

6

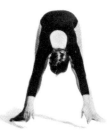

Traditional Exercises and Why They Don't Work

You may have noticed that there are some well known exercises that aren't included in this book. That's because *The Tummy Trimmer Primer* consists of a group of exercises specially designed to reduce the stomach and hips through the principle of the uplifted body and the open stretch line. Other exercises aren't part of that concept.

The omission of the bicycle exercise in particular, in which you lie on your back and push up the legs and lower body for the purpose of pedaling in the air, is worth noting. So many people do it, thinking it's good for something. But the tendency is to concentrate on the pedaling action of the legs while the whole bulk of your torso is allowed to sag.

If any value were to be had from that exercise, it would only come from reaching your toes for the ceiling as high as possible in order to keep the weight off your hips. The pedaling should be slow with deliberately pointed toes, and concentration should be on stretching your feet toward the ceiling so that your stomach muscles are held in check and the muscle tone tightened.

Some people use stationary bicycle machines thinking they're doing themselves some good, but there again, the tendency is to concentrate on the pedaling action of the legs, allowing the rest of the body to sit immobile on the seat.

If any value were to be had from stationary bicycling, it would only come from pedaling with reciprocal muscle action going through the entire torso. Most children ride bicycles that way naturally; it seems to be in tune with their growing pattern. Why stop the total body involvement when growth has stopped? Yet when you see an adult riding a bicycle, or sitting atop a machine, you usually only see spinning legs.

If you like the bicycle exercise and want to keep doing it, make sure you push through your whole body instead of just wildly pedaling your legs. The same advice holds if you have a bicycle machine. But even better advice is to do the real thing if possible.

The process involved in bicycle riding is one which unifies the whole body. Your legs begin the action and your torso and arms become involved in moving and controlling the bicycle. When one foot is up, the other is down and so each leg becomes alternately active and passive as the body moves forward with alternating activity and rest going on in the rest of the body at the same time. You then have horizontal movement as a result of vertical effort.

This is total muscular teamwork operating on a unifying line through the whole body. It's an excellent example of the same proportioning line I've been describing throughout this book, put into recreational action. You can find similar benefit in any recreational exercise you choose.

Every recreational exercise has its own style, but the basic action is all the same—total body exercise which includes the mind and satisfies the emotions. You can find it in bowling; you can find it in croquet. Get out there and have a little fun in your spare time instead of sitting around growing a large stomach and hips.

7

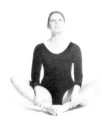

Staying Trim

It isn't necessary to list all the ways you can exercise, as long as you carry the uplift concept with you. Whether you try archery, badminton, calisthenics, dancing, fencing, fishing, gardening, gymnastics, handball, hang gliding, hiking, ice skating, judo, karate, paddle tennis, sailing, swimming, table tennis, T'ai Chi Ch'uan, or any of the other things I forgot to list doesn't matter; it's your choice. Whatever you choose and enjoy is right for you and your body.

But we all walk, and *every* place we go we take our bodies along with us—mostly in horizontal movement, but sometimes altered to include the verticals presented by stairs, curbs, or ramps, with all the pauses, hesitations, accelerations, and decelerations of tempo within the movement. Walking causes shifting of body weights, levels, and planes and that constant adjustment that threatens our uplifted posture.

It's easy to take for granted the actual process of walking, easy also to ignore a responsibility to the body parts in walking and just how they need to be carried.

There are fifty-two little bones in the feet that make it possible for us to walk. They should make ground contact with the heels and balls of the feet, and your weight should be evenly distributed between them. If the body weight is allowed to pitch toward the arches, it can throw the entire body skeleton out of alignment, sabotaging the carriage of the upper body. Ideally, the upper body should stay high, keeping the weight up and avoiding any pitch in the ankles that would affect the arches.

If you have been a person whose excess weight has shifted down to your waistline, weakened the pelvic muscles, and forced your stomach out and enlarged your hips, and you've also had a misalignment coming up from your feet, you have had a real bulge clash going on. There has been no place for that poor stomach to go but out to the front.

So you've got to be thinking of that invisible axis of perfect alignment as you walk—the line from your head through the chest and pelvis, from which everything is supposed to operate successfully in its proper place. You've got to pay attention to the straightness of your body not only standing and sitting but also in walking.

It's easy to do, especially now that you understand the uplift concept. All you have to do is inhale, raise your eye level and the tilt of your chin, and away you go.

What actually happens when you walk is that your weight falls forward through all the body joints, is controlled by centering muscles, and is met by the alternating leg swinging forward to catch your weight and support it while the pattern repeats itself. There's a pendulum effect as the legs swing from the hip sockets, and any tension that's accumulated from the muscle fatigue of standing or sitting still for a long time is released. All this goes on without your thinking about it.

But if you want to think a bit as you walk, you have a great opportunity to practice and improve your stomach control so that you can maintain its flatness and keep the extra weight from settling in your hips.

Notice that when you stop your gait (especially suddenly) there's an automatic stomach muscle tightening that takes place. It also happens when you step down from a curb and up again on the other side of a street.

Every time that happens, tighten it a little more, releasing, but not letting go as you resume your gait. And when you step up the curb, or go up steps, use the stomach muscles as the motivating force to lift your feet rather than letting your knees assume all the action and letting your legs bear more body weight than they need to.

In walking, the process of losing your balance and quickly recovering it causes less strain than the effort needed to keep your body in one position. When you stand still you have to keep all your equilibrium in one place and that takes more energy. That's why people pace the floor instead of standing motionless in periods of stress; instinct helps them preserve their energy and make it last for the duration of their stress.

Night walking is easier and quieter than day walking because you don't have so many visual distractions. You automatically return to the old primary patterns of movement that aren't so affected by self-conscious reactions, and the body is completely free to relax and restore itself. (Nightwalking in unsafe areas, of course, has the opposite effect.)

Walking is good for you. It's a steady, natural, rhythmic pattern of movement that can keep your whole body in tune, soothe it, and amuse your mind at the same time. It's especially pleasant when you don't have to carry a big stomach and large hips around with you.

Give your walk a lift so it will, in turn, give you a lift because staying uplifted is what being in shape is all about.

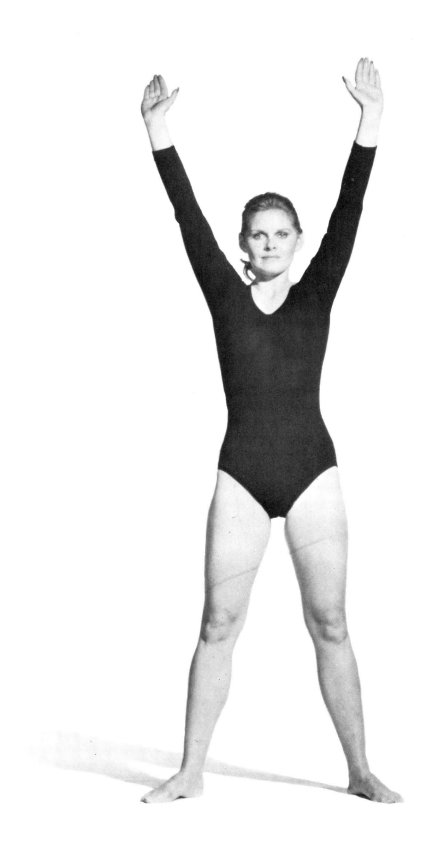

Index

T

W